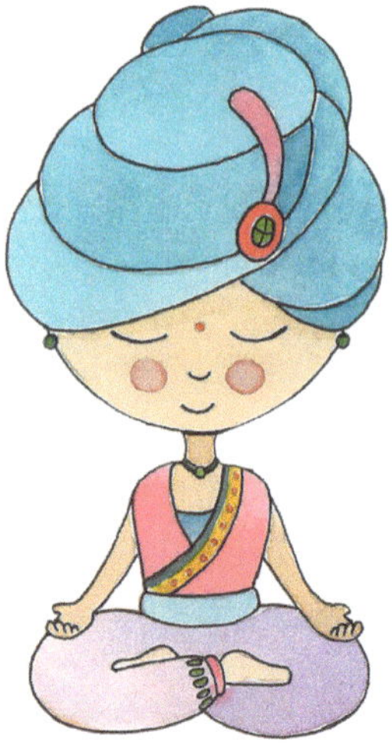

THE LITTLE PRINCE OF YOGA

By: Melissa Ferrer

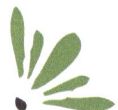

For my son **Pietro Alessandro**.

Thank you to all my guiding forces.
May all beings be free and happy.

Special thanks to Giacomo Salizzoni.

Melissa Ferrer
Author/Creator

Angelique Colte
Illustrator

Mk Angeles
Graphic Designer

Hello!

Mukha Svansana
(downward facing dog)

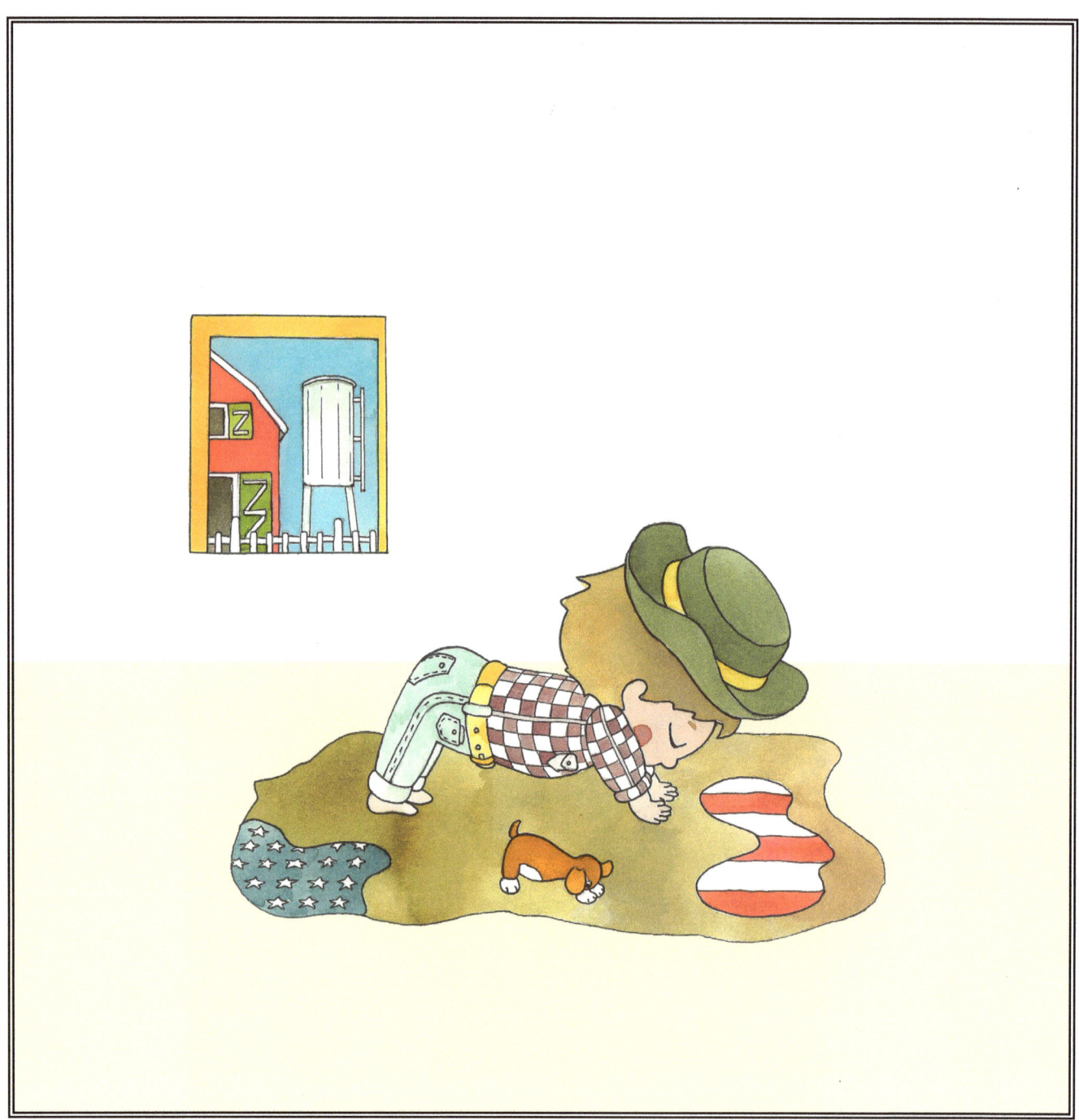

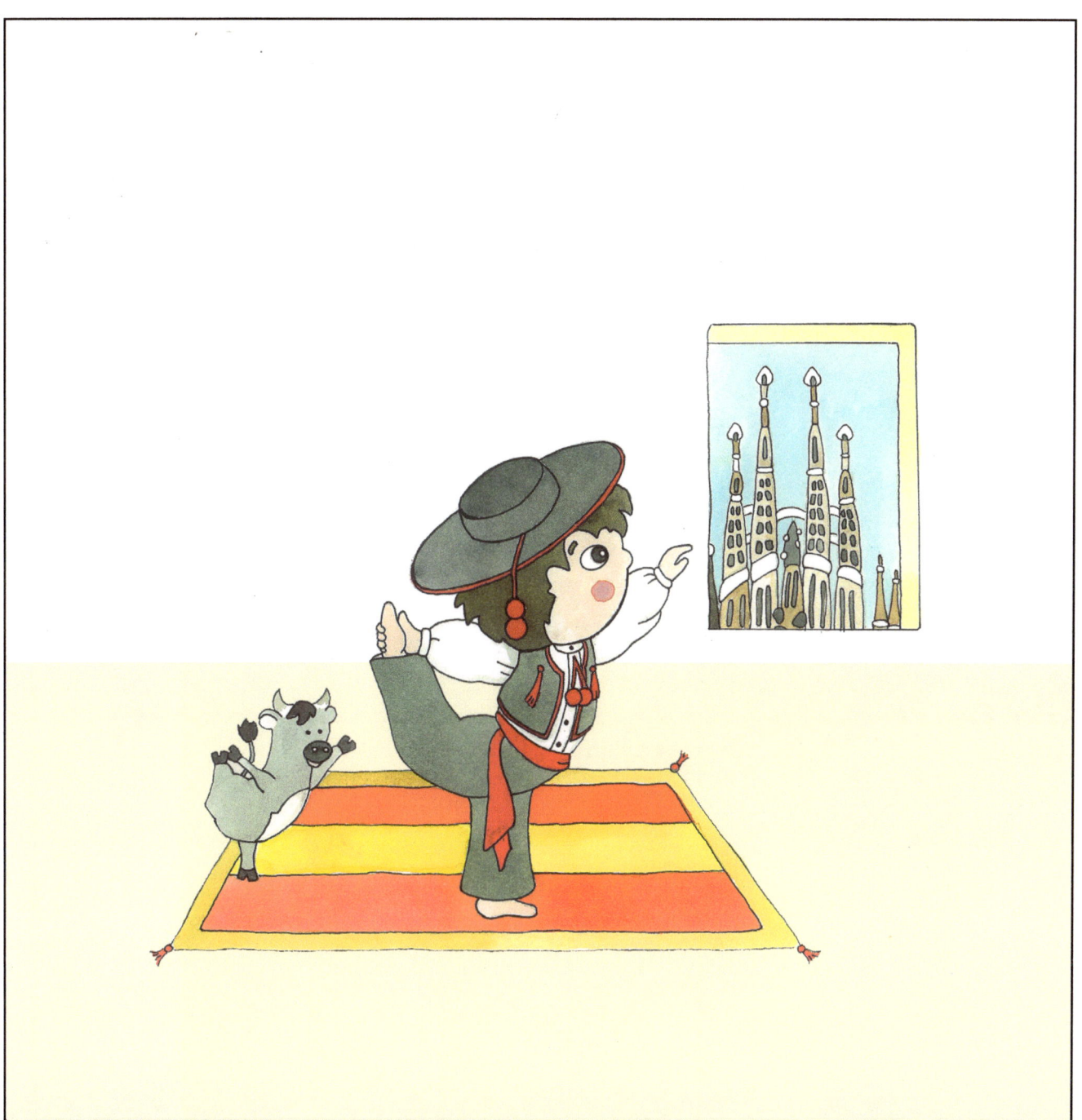

¡Hola!

Natarajasana
(dancer's pose)

¡Buenos días!

Vrksasana

(tree pose)

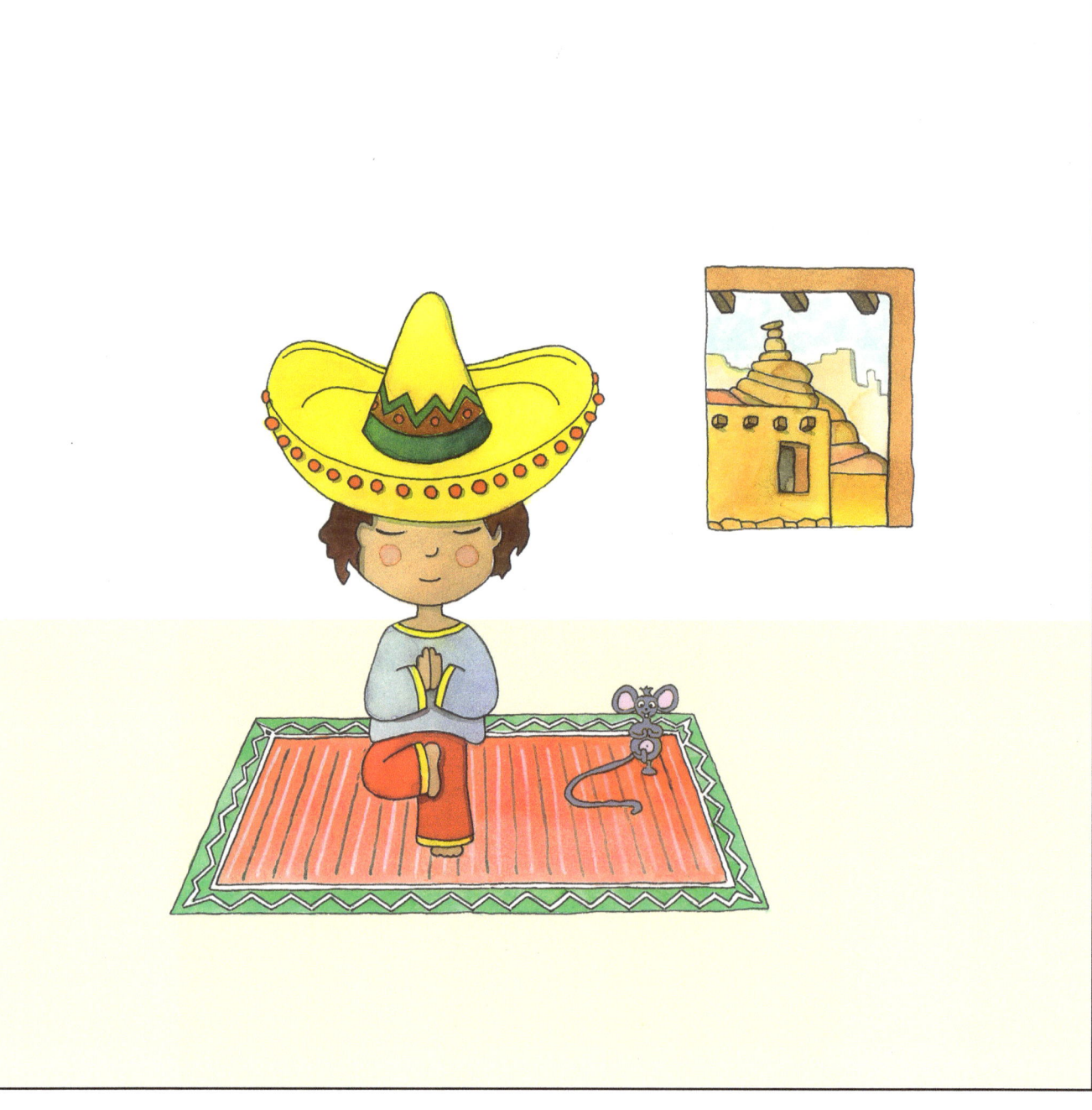

Ciao!

Setu Bandha Sarvangasana

(modified bridge pose)

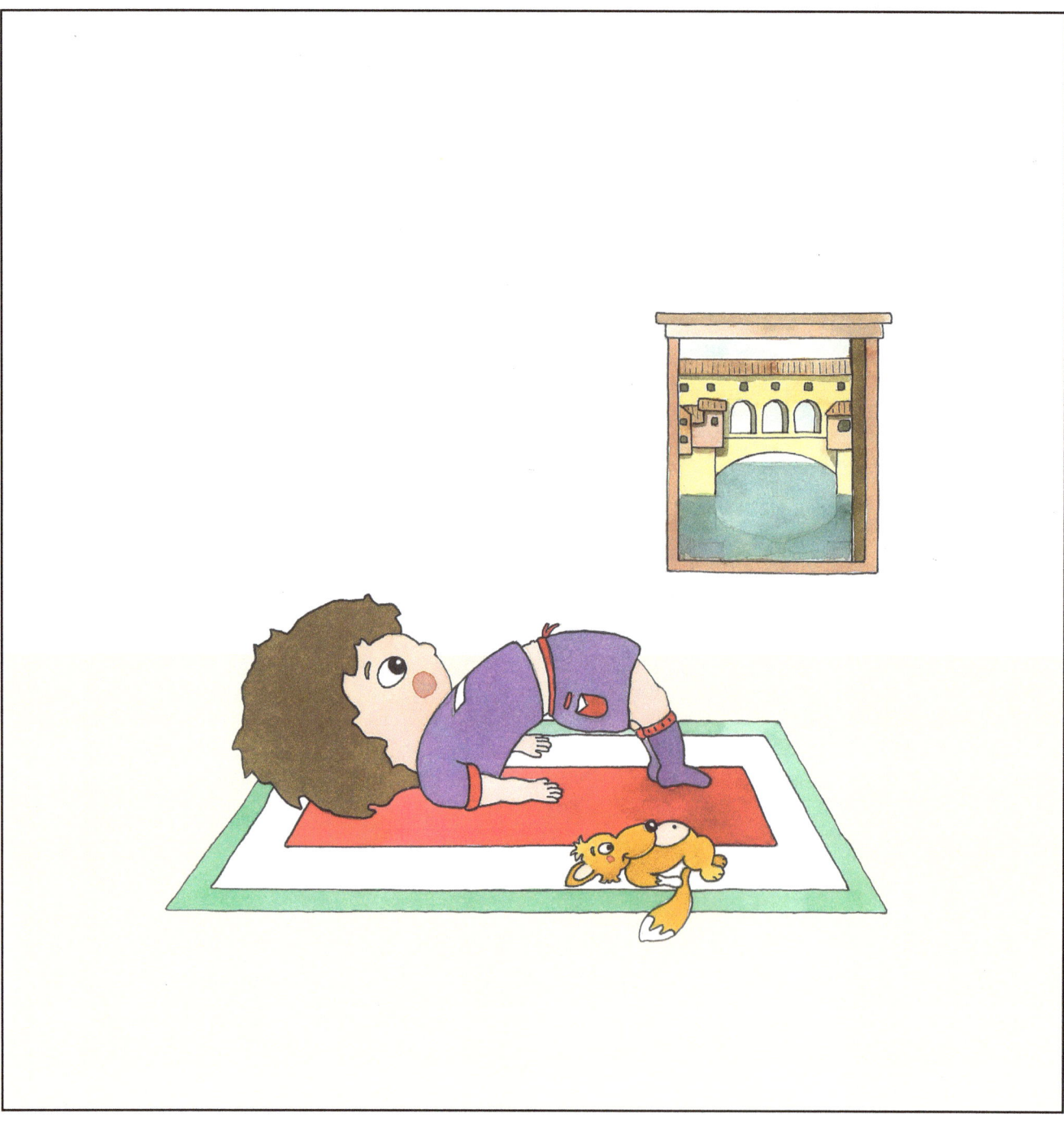

Hello!

Urdhva Mukha Svanasana

(upward facing dog)

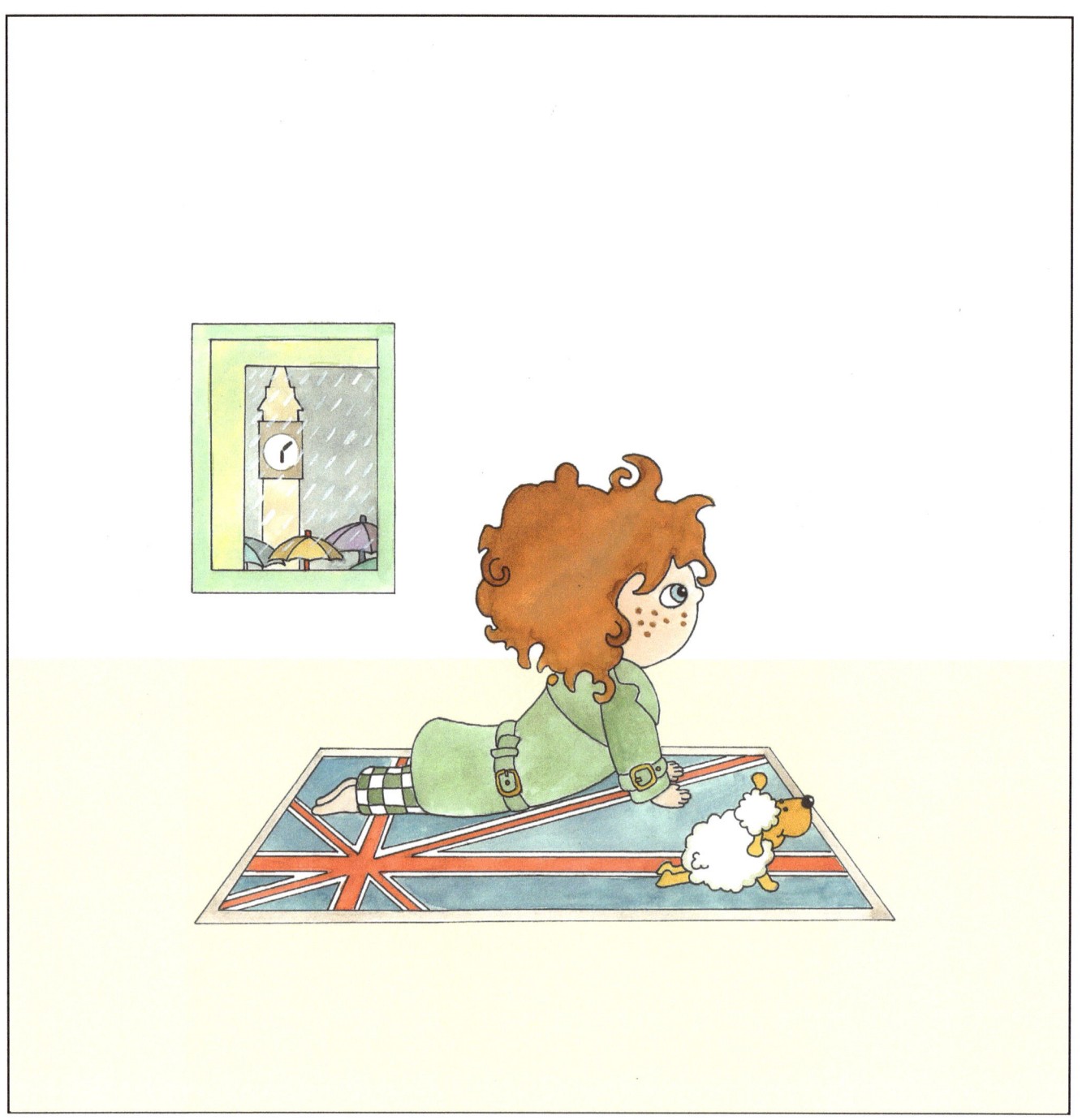

Namaste!

Padmasana

(lotus)

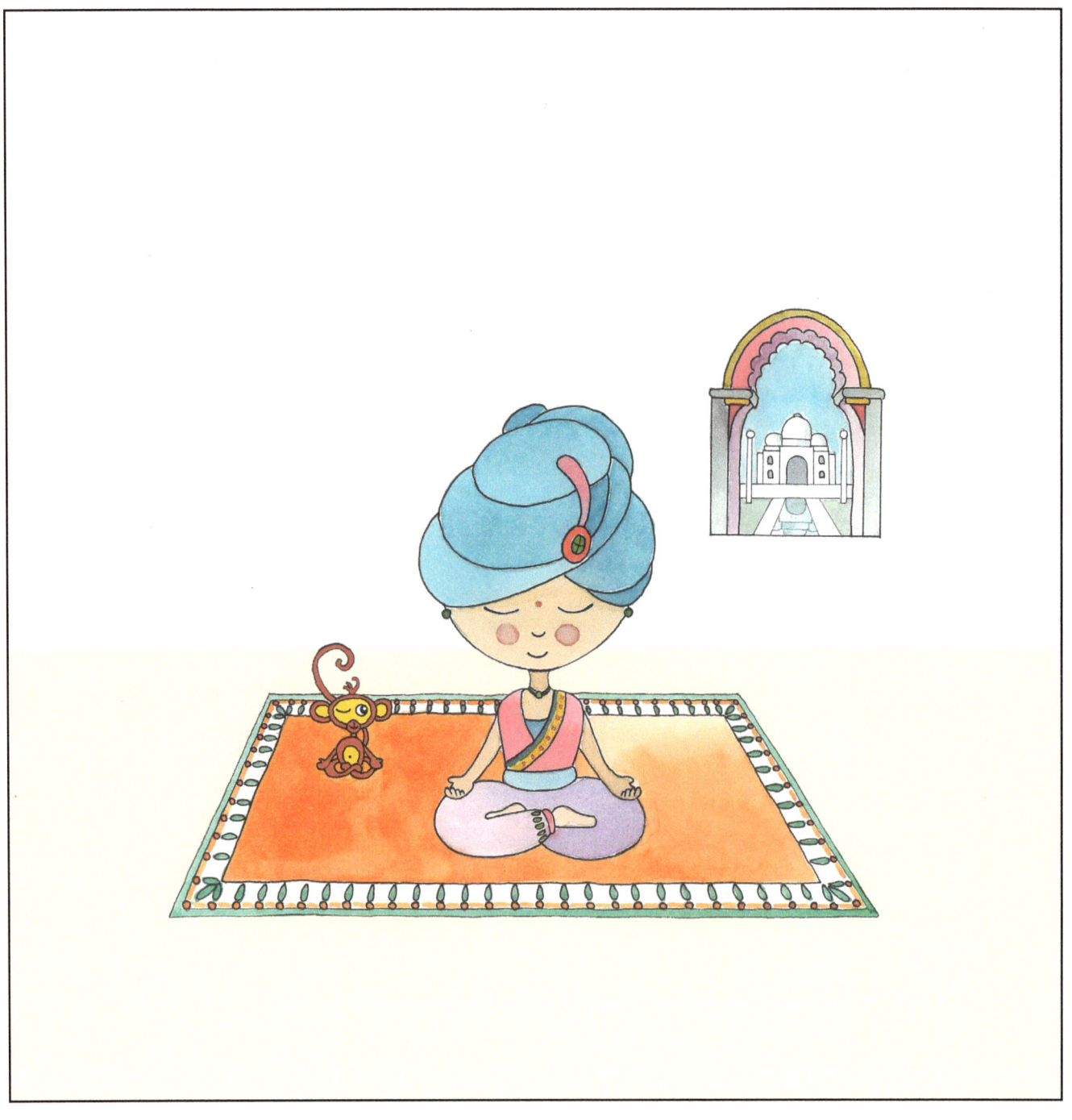

Konnichiwa!

Virabhadrasana I

(warrior pose I)

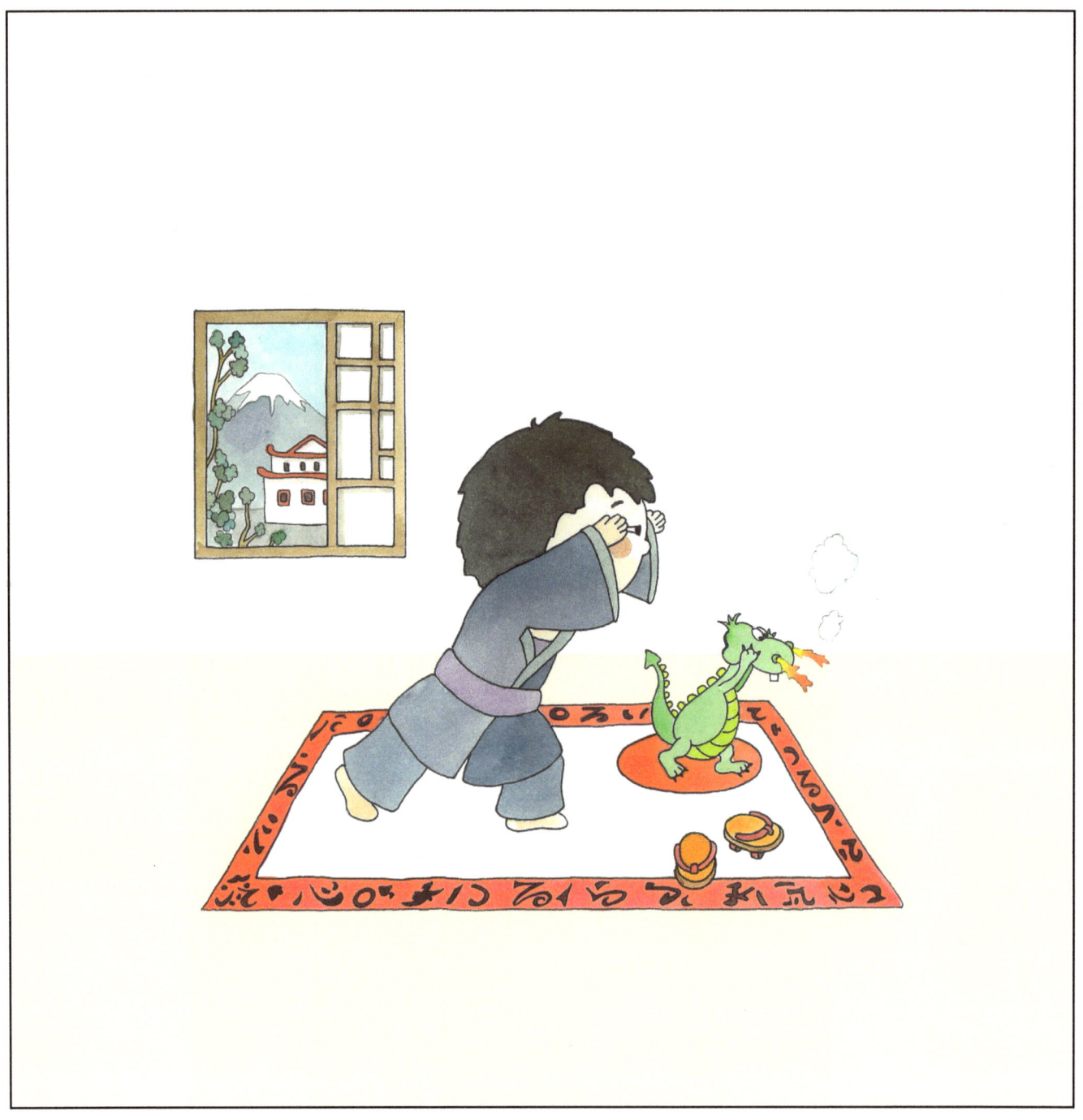

Bonjour!

Parivrtta Trikonasana

(revolved triangle pose)

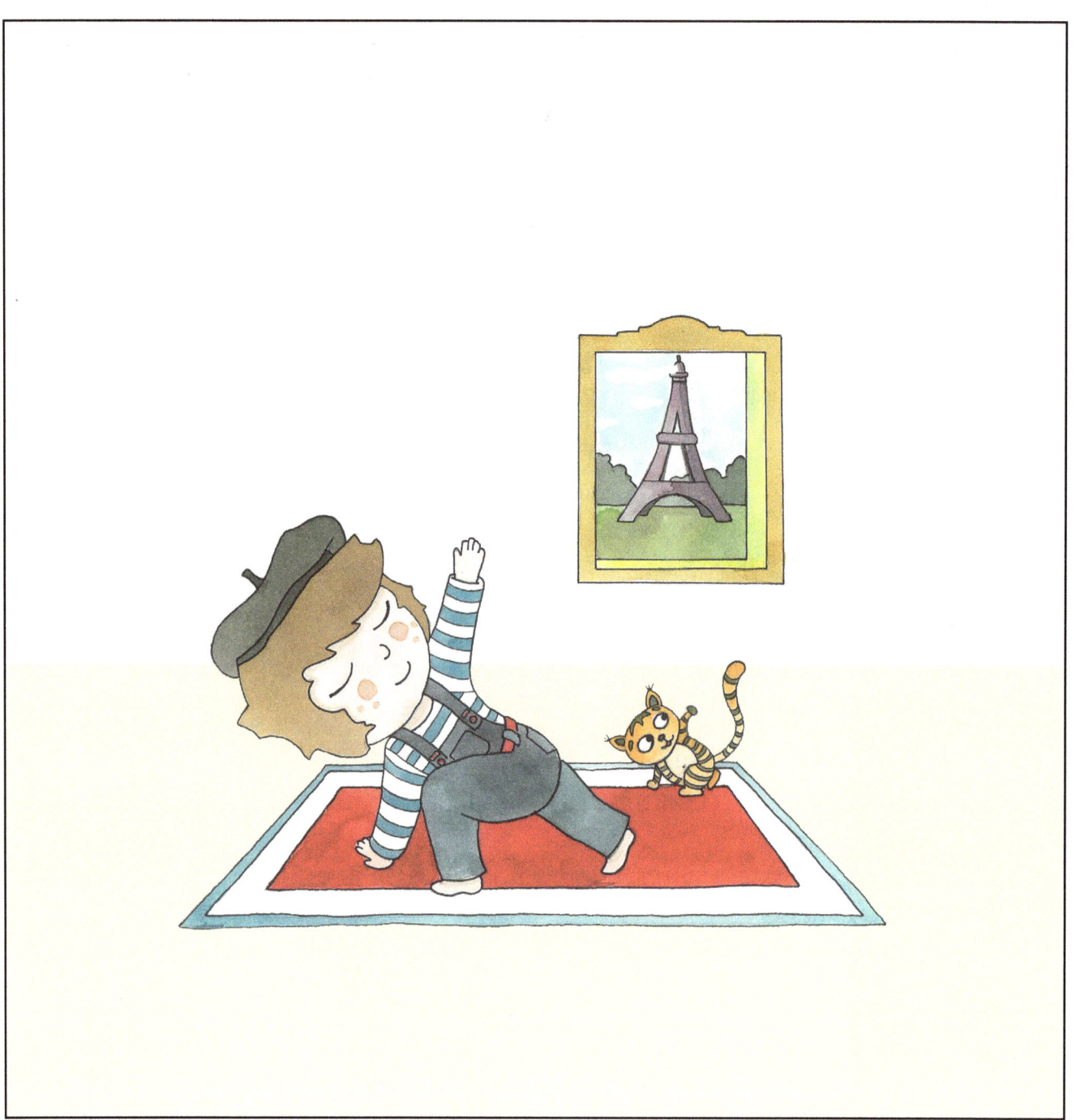

Ni Hao!

Virabhadrasana II
(warrior pose II)

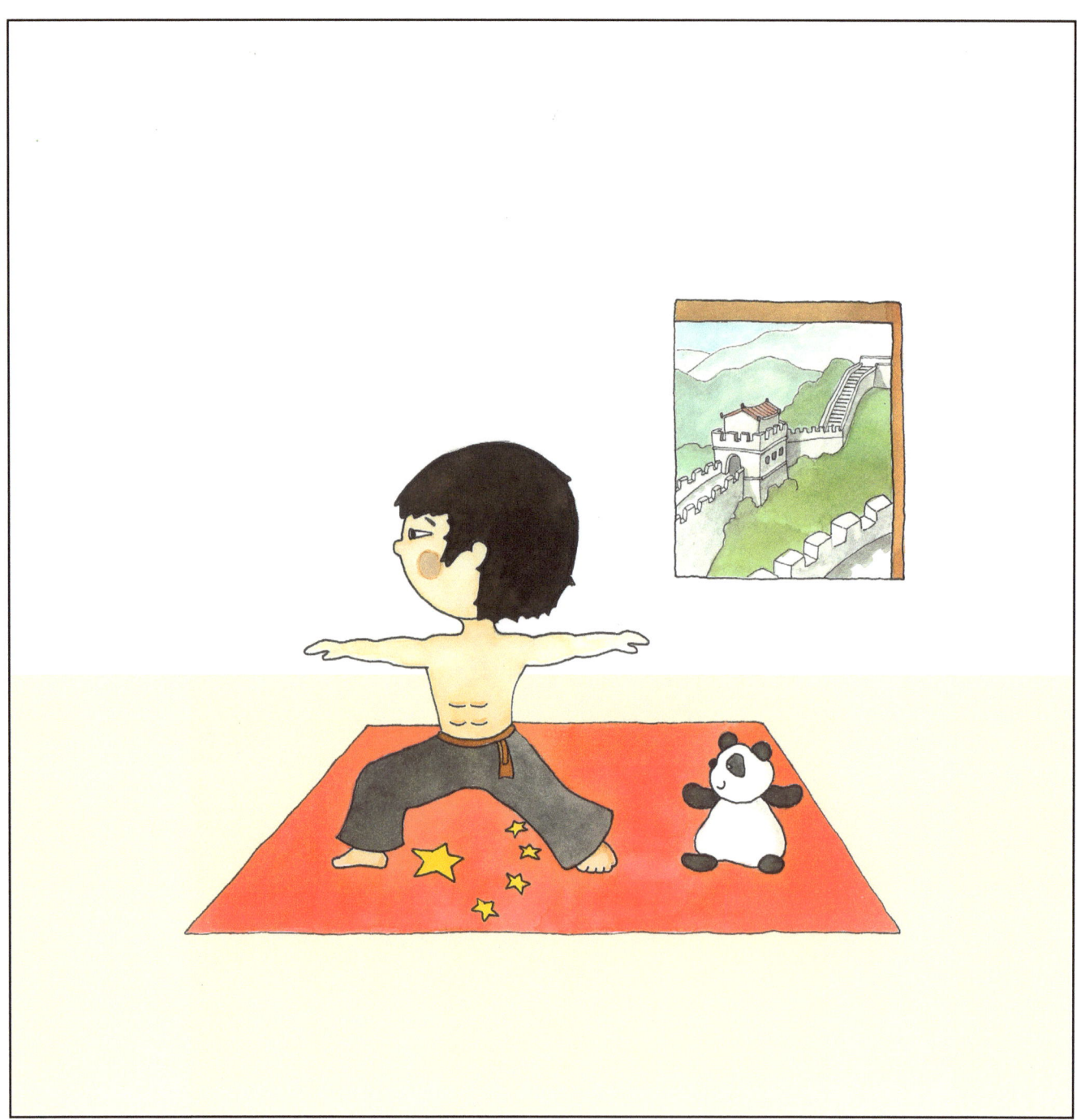

Olá!

Bakasana

(crow pose)

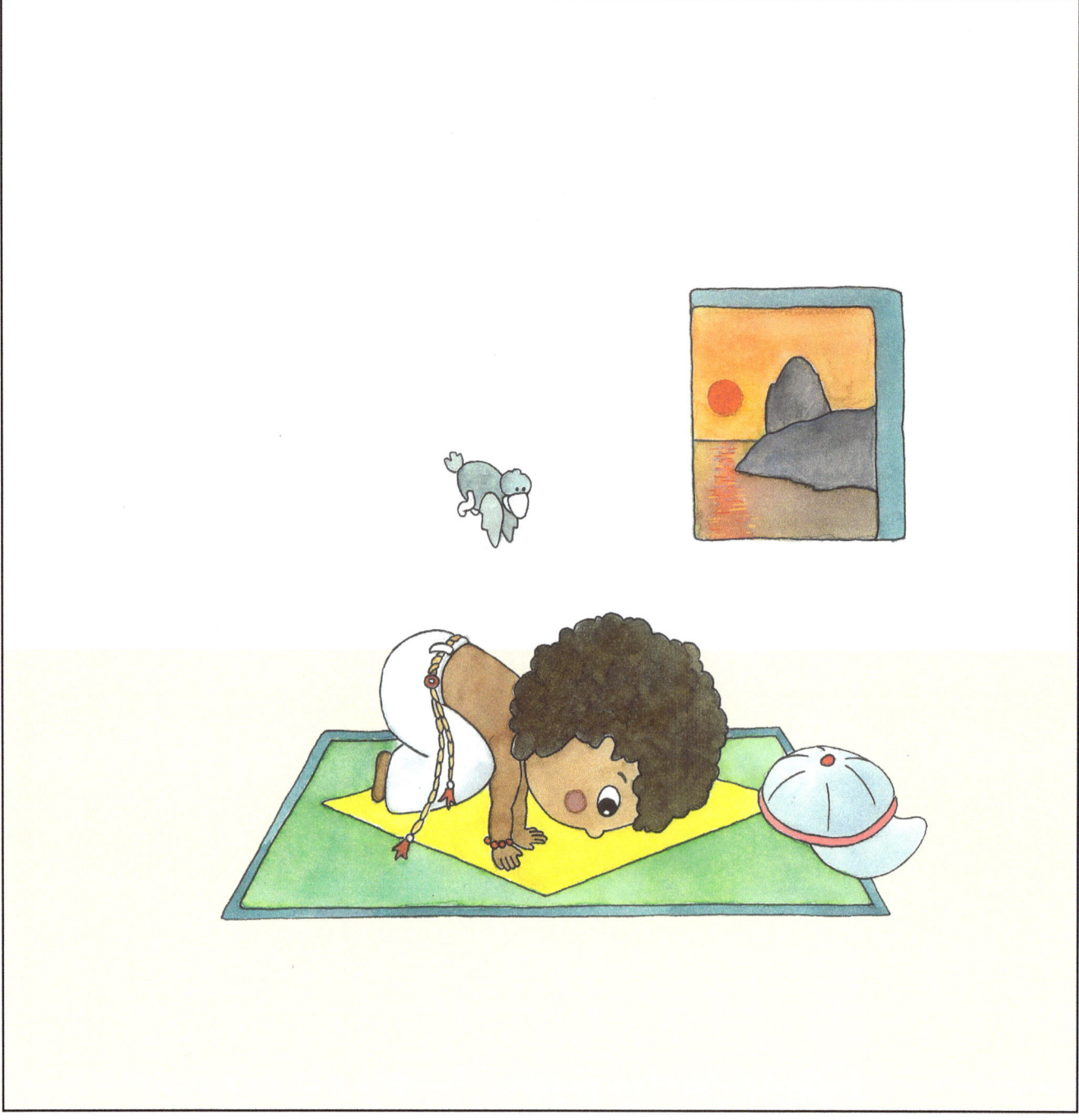

Haai!

Utkatasana

(fierce pose)

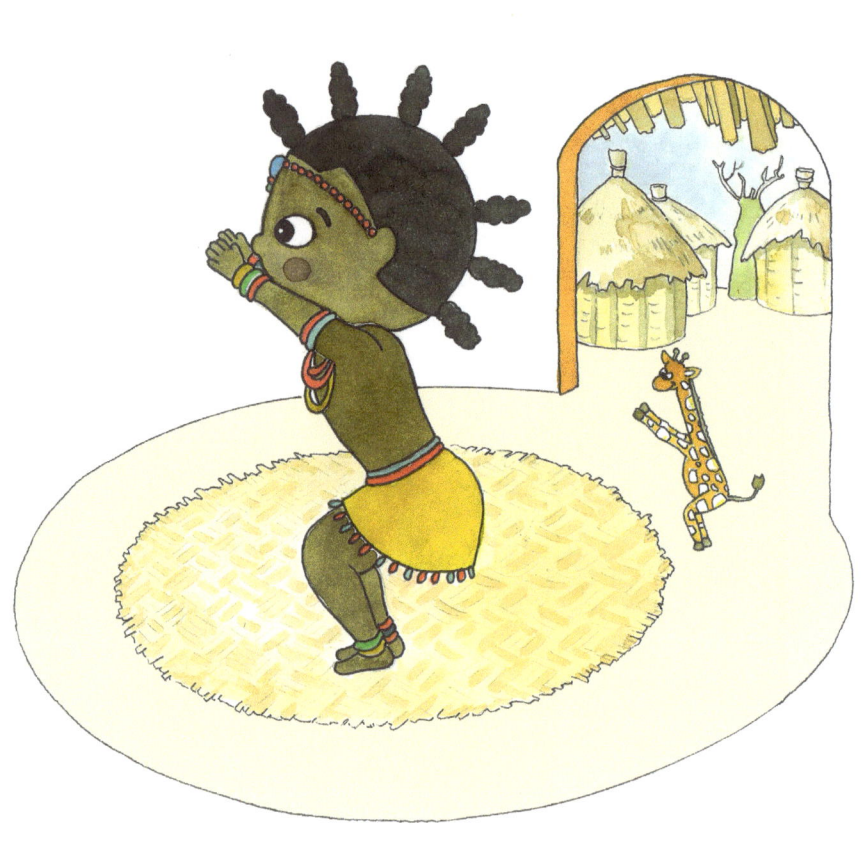

Privet!

Sirsha-asana
(head-stand pose)

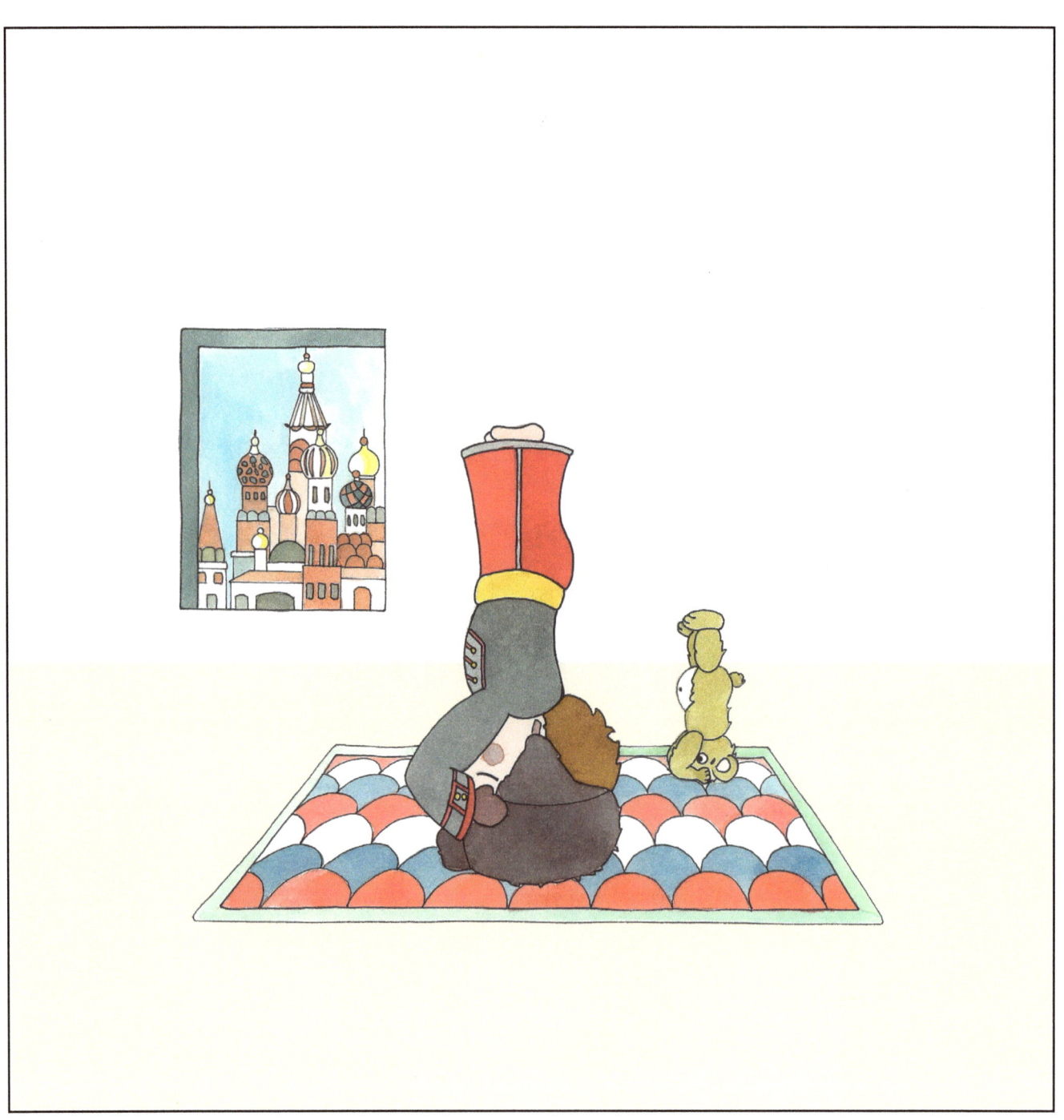

Closing Prayer

स्वस्तिप्रजाभ्यः परिपालयंतां न्यायेन मार्गेण महीं महीशाः ।
गोब्राह्मणेभ्यः शुभमस्तु नित्यं लोकासमस्ता सुखिनोभवंतु ॥

May all be well with mankind.
May the leaders of the earth protect
in every way by keeping the right path.

May there be goodness for all those
who know the earth to be sacred.
May all worlds be happy.

About The Author

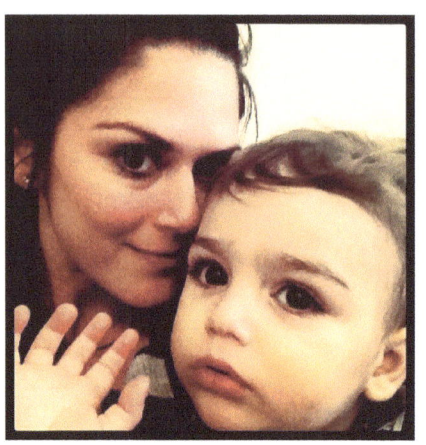

Melissa Ferrer- Salizzoni was born and raised in Miami, Florida. She has trained over 500 hours in Ashtanga yoga throughout San Francisco, Puerto Rico and Stockholm. This practice her helped her grow both physically and mentally strong. Her fitness background includes core training, Pilates and gymnastics. She owns 19r Yoga & Pilates in Florence, Italy and co-owns Yoga to Go Vacations, leading seasonal retreats all over the world.

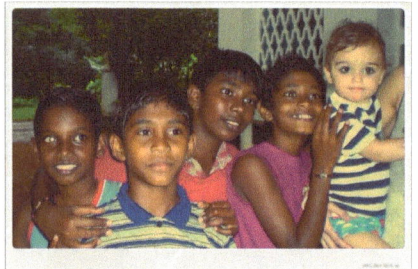

A portion of proceeds from "The Little Prince of Yoga" goes to Christian Society of India located in Kerala, India. The all boys orphanage provides support and education to school age children in the South West of Kerala.

www.melissayoga.net
www.19ryogapilates.com
www.yogatogovacations.com

Melissa@19ryogapilates.com

www.ingramcontent.com/pod-product-compliance
Lightning Source LLC
Chambersburg PA
CBHW040308010626
45792CB00025B/1480